Bipolar Disorder: A Journey from Darkness to Acceptance

J.L Douglas

Published by ebook worm publishing, 2024.

BIPOLAR DISORDER: A JOURNEY FROM DARKNESS TO ACCEPTANCE

First edition. March 25, 2024.

Copyright © 2024 J.L Douglas.

ISBN: 979-8224595211

Written by J.L Douglas.

or its affiliates, in the Unites States and other countries and may not be used without written permission. All other trademarks are the property of their respective owners. eBook Work Publishing is not associated with any products or vendor mentioned in this book.

BIPOLAR DISORDER: A JOURNEY FROM DARKNESS TO ACCEPTANCE.

CHAPTER 1

INTRODUCTION

The humid Georgia summer of 1998 clung to me like a damp blanket, oppressive and inescapable. The empty house closed in on me with an ominous silence as I aimlessly wandered from room to room. I jumped at every creak and groan of the old floorboards settling; my frayed nerves wound tight. The rare solitude should have been peaceful with the boys at a friend's house. Instead, the quite reverberated, amplifying my anxiety.

I couldn't take it anymore. I started scrubbing the already impeccable kitchen furiously as if I could scour away the unease taking hold. I ruthlessly attacked each surface, pouring my agitated mind into the mindless task. As I vigorously wiped the gleaming appliances, I caught my reflection in the chrome finish. A tense, wild-eyed woman I barely recognized stared back at me.

When every inch shone spotlessly, I collapsed onto the couch, limp with exhaustion. But almost immediately, I was up again, pacing restlessly as foreboding pressed down on me. I felt the ominous approach of some nameless catastrophe that lurked just out of view, soon to rupture my world.

I tried to push away the paranoid thoughts, telling myself I was letting my imagination run wild. But I couldn't ignore the prickling dread needling under my skin. The empty house held sinister shadows that I swore wavered at the corner of my vision. I whirled around but found nothing.

A glance at the clock told me it was past midnight, but I knew there was no point trying to sleep. Nonetheless, I finally passed out fully dressed on the lumpy couch, too drained to make it upstairs to bed.

As I slipped in and out of unsettling dreams, I endlessly opened doors down shadowy corridors, fruitlessly searching room after empty room for someone I couldn't find. Faceless figures lingered just out of view, always disappearing when I turned. I strained to hear a distant voice calling me urgently, needing my help. But I made no progress through the endless maze, no matter how hard I ran. Trapped in a twisted limbo, I couldn't escape.

I jolted awake to the sound of a loud crack splitting the silence. I lay frozen, heart pounding out of my chest, ears straining. After endless minutes of silence, I started to calm down. Settling house, that's all. But no sooner had I taken a deep breath than another splintering bang vibrated through the room. I whimpered, drawing my knees to my chest. This couldn't just be the old building. No, my gut told me this had to be the nameless catastrophe I had sensed approaching...now arriving to violently rupture my world without warning.

I sat rigid, listening raptly, but heard nothing aside from my jagged breathing. An hour must have passed before I could force myself to stand on shaky legs to inspect all the doors and windows. My pulse hammered in my ears as I checked each lock, affirming everything was secured tight, undisturbed. But an ominous feeling still needled me. That cracking had been a bone-chilling warning of impending disaster.

Exhausted and rattled, I sank back onto the lumpy couch as the first glow of dawn lit the living room. The pale light pushed back the murky shadows I imagined creeping along the walls. As my adrenaline finally ebbed, my thoughts slowed. You have to get it together – for the boys, at least. It was just an old house settling. Nothing sinister.

But no amount of rational lecturing could ease the pit in my stomach or halt the paranoid visions flickering through my mind. Something sinister lurked just out of sight; I could feel its relentless approach in the tingling of my skin.

I must have dozed off because suddenly, I was jolted violently, alert by an explosion of splintering cracks vibrating through the walls. I leaped up in sheer terror, convinced the entire house was about to come crashing down around me.

But an endless stretch of deafening silence followed. There was no crumbling of walls, no intruders breaking through locked doors.

Tentatively, I made another complete circuit of the house, checking for damage or anything amiss. Again, I found nothing. Only my footprints tracking back and forth across the floors indicated movement.

Nonetheless, I couldn't dispel the chilling sense that this was the crisis I had sensed approaching...now arriving to rupture everything without warning.

I huddled on the couch, watching the minutes tick by, ears straining. But aside from the pounding of my own heart, only silence echoed through the rooms. The walls remained intact. Early dawn light filtered through the undamaged windows. The front door stood closed, the porch empty. By all appearances, everything was as it should be.

Yet unease still flooded my veins like ice. Indeed, that splintering crack felt too violent to be just the old building settling, the first herald of disaster. I strained into the silence, jumping at the slightest sounds. The thudding refrigerator kicking on made me yelp. The groaning pipe valves created bursts of adrenaline. I stared wide-eyed into dim corners, braced for shadows to take monstrous shapes before my eyes. But nothing transformed except in my increasingly frenzied thoughts.

Dawn gave way to early morning outside - songbirds trilled under a hazy blue sky. Another typically peaceful Sunday morning in our quiet neighborhood. I watched a couple of families leaving for church, my neighbors' laughter floating faintly through the window as they loaded kids into minivans. Their benign normalcy taunted me as I sat paralyzed.

Suddenly, I wondered if I was losing my grip on reality. Perhaps I had imagined the whole incident after another primarily sleepless night. It wouldn't be the first vivid waking dream conjured by exhaustion and anxiety. But even as I desperately tried to reassure myself, I had hallucinated the vivid sensory details, I knew deep down this had been different. The shuddering cracks had originated from outside my troubled mind and uneasy imagination.

But if not a delusion or nightmare, then what? As the morning approached midday, nothing else occurred inside or outside the still house. By early afternoon, the mundane reality of neighbors mowing lawns and walking dogs steadily eroded the vivid memories of violence cracking open my early morning. Could it have been some freak, strange incident I imagined more meaning into? As the hours without further incident slowly ticked, I cautiously allowed my heartbeat to decelerate toward normal rhythms.

Until that is, I was violently dragged back into high alert by another jagged crack blasting through the wall behind me, seemingly shaking the very foundation beneath my feet. I cried out before clamping my hand over my mouth, heart jackhammering against my ribs, fully expecting the entire structure to start splintering and crumbling around me. I squeezed my eyes shut, waiting for the impact of shattering glass and caving walls...

But again, no collapse came. After endless frozen minutes, I tentatively cracked my eyes open again. Everything looked unchanged, innocuously normal. The pale-yellow living room walls stood intact, dusty rays of midafternoon light slanting across faded upholstery. The front door remained closed; the heavy silence broken only by the rapid pace of my breathing.

CHAPTER 2

THE ONSET

I huddled on the couch; knees pulled tight to my chest as the disembodied cracking reverberated through the walls again. Heart slamming against my ribs, I squeezed my eyes shut, willing it all to go away.

Just an old house settling, I repeated desperately in my head. But the sinister booming seemed to mock me, heralding my worst fears brought to life.

When the next resounding crack split the air, I couldn't take it. I leaped up, the room tilting around me. I had to get out of here. I grabbed my purse and keys blindly and stumbled to the front door on leaden legs.

The pre-dawn August air clung to me, already humid and oppressive. In the eerie stillness, the uneven thud of my footsteps on the pavement seemed unnaturally loud. At the edge of the porch, I froze. Some rational part of my mind screamed that it wasn't safe out here alone, urging me to return inside. But being trapped in that house under the mercy of the unseen threat overpowered logic.

With shaking hands, I fumbled the car door open before peeling out onto the street, the houses blurring past in the gloom. The empty road spooled out before me as I sped up, my harsh breathing and pounding pulse thundering in my ears. Dark woods flanked the road on both sides, shadows rising to consume me.

A fragment of a half-remembered Bible verse about the valley of the shadow of death rose in my mind. I tried to blink it away, desperately groping for rational thought, but the shadows only loomed darker.

Suddenly, I slammed on the brakes, the tires screeching in protest. A massive oak precariously hung over the road as if teetering on the verge of toppling directly onto my car. I threw the vehicle into reverse, the branches seeming to scrape the roof as I tore backward.

Finally, a gap wide enough to squeeze through appeared, and I gunned the gas pedal. The car lurched back onto the open road as I gasped for air, my ragged breath echoing.

In some distant recess of my mind, an inner voice argued weakly that it was just a fallen tree, not a malicious entity deliberately blocking my path. But now that the terror had me in its grip, it would not loosen its hold. A cacophony of disjointed thoughts careened through my brain, slamming into each other with the force of a multi-car pileup. I was at the wheel of a runaway vehicle I could not control.

As I sped on, the headlights tunneled a feeble path through the impenetrable darkness. Suddenly, they glinted off reflective eyes on the shoulder of the road just ahead. I swerved wildly to avoid the deer frozen directly in my path, nearly driving into the ditch before wrestling the steering wheel back under control.

My chest heaved as I choked back sobs, hands shaking violently against the wheel. Still, I pushed the gas pedal down further, tires humming against the pavement. I had no destination, only the panicked, primal need to outrun real and imagined dangers.

Suddenly, flashing lights appeared in my rearview mirror, the siren slicing through my fog. Some remaining shred of rationality recognized the familiar markings of a police car, but the instinctual fear response prevailed.

I accelerated still faster as the sirens wailed. The terror of pulling over and being trapped inside the vehicle overpowered any logical thought of obeying the police. A voice boomed through a megaphone, distorted and inhuman, commanding me to stop. I hunched lower over the wheel, hair whipping wildly around my face.

I rounded a curve at breakneck speed, barely keeping the car on the road. The sirens faded briefly as the flashing lights disappeared from view. Up ahead, I spotted a weathered barn and veered sharply towards it on impulse, skidding to a precarious stop just inside.

My breath came in ragged, raw gasps as I scrambled from the car and stumbled more deeply into the musty dimness. Somewhere in the recesses of my consciousness, I registered the absurdity of hiding here like a fugitive, but self-preservation overpowered reason.

Crouched in a corner behind rusty, abandoned equipment, I made myself as small as possible. Every tiny sound magnified in my ears—the scurrying of mice in the walls, the creak of rafters overhead. It all blurred with my panicked wheezing until I could no longer distinguish the noise source.

After endless, frantic minutes when no one appeared, my taut, trembling muscles began to unlock slightly. With weak legs, I pulled myself to my feet, edging towards the dingy window to peer out. An empty driveway and dark, silent woods were all that greeted me. No police lights flashing, no impending doom waiting to consume me.

I nearly sobbed in relief, leaning heavily against the rough wood wall as my knees threatened to give way. The morning light had fully crept over the landscape, burnishing everything in a deceptively warm glow. I could almost pretend it had all been a twisted nightmare for a moment.

But as I turned shakily towards the car, reality came crashing back in full force. The events of the past hours had been all too real. I had no idea where I was or how I would get home.

Panic reared up again at the thought. I couldn't stay at this abandoned farm, yet I was in no state to drive or face the police if they caught up to me. An anguished cry wrenched from my throat as I looked desperately around for answers that would not materialize.

Suddenly, my eyes landed on an old tractor at the rear of the barn. Without pausing to consider the absurdity of my actions, I hurried over and climbed up to hide in the seat behind the steering wheel. My knees curled to my chest; I made myself as small as possible. If anyone found me now, I indeed looked utterly deranged.

But I could not stop the childlike instinct to hide. I had to be concealed from the danger, tucked safely away where the looming threats could not find me. Logic and reason had long since deserted me, leaving only primal panic and fear.

I have no idea how long I remained sealed in that tractor cab. Time lost all meaning, minutes bleeding into hours in a nightmarish limbo state. Cramps radiated through my torso from the clenched, unyielding position, but still, I did not - could not - move.

I flinched violently at the sudden sound of a vehicle approaching outside. Had they come for me at last? Fresh waves of panic crashed over me as floorboards creaked under approaching footsteps. This was it - I had nowhere left to run or hide. I closed my eyes as though I might somehow remain concealed by not seeing my pursuers.

"Elisa?" A tentative but familiar voice filtered through the heavy door. My head snapped up. Larry? Before I could process this development, the door swung open, revealing my friend's kind face creased in concern.

Disbelief flooded me. Larry lived nearly an hour away - how had he possibly found me here? But coherent questions could not push through the tangled chaos in my brain.

I opened my mouth but only managed a strangled sob. Gently, patiently, Larry coaxed me down from the tractor seat, keeping up a soothing murmur as if comforting a wounded animal. I leaned heavily against him, limp with the relief of being found. Being saved, though I did not fully understand what.

My memory of the drive back blurs into fragments - street signs and storefronts flashing past while I hunched in the passenger seat, Larry's steady voice navigating me back from the ledge of reality. navigated by the time he pulled in at the small local hospital, the world had ceased tilting quite violently. But I still felt anchored outside myself, present in body but detached in mind.

Larry kept a steadying hand on my elbow as we navigated the bright halls that seemed garish to my shell-shocked senses. There were forms placed in front of me that I dutifully signed without comprehending.

Then, the chill of a stethoscope against my back, the pressure of a blood pressure cuff squeezing my arm like a vise. I complied woodenly with each new procedure, too numb to feel fear or question.

At some point, a petite nurse took my arm, gently guiding me away from Larry and towards a stark room. Though every fiber of my being cried out to resist, some instinct forced me to put one foot in front of the other until we reached the bare space to be my new refuge. Or was it my prison cell? The distinction blurred in my fractured mind.

The door closed behind me with an echoing thud of finality, the lock turning with an ominous click. I took in the room with wild eyes - simple bed, plastic chair, a small window through which morning light filtered, casting bars of shadow across the floor. The image wavered before me edges shifting in and out of blurred focus. Or perhaps reality had ceased adhering to any natural laws, leaving me adrift in an unmoored world. On weak legs, I stumbled to the bed, collapsing as the last of my manic energy seeped away. As I stared at the blank ceiling tiles, the events replayed like some horrific movie montage. Had that been me tearing through the night, hiding like a hunted creature in an abandoned barn? Or had I crossed into some nightmarish alternate reality where my worst fears played out for sadistic entertainment?

Perhaps if I closed my eyes tight enough, I would wake up back in my bed to find it had all been a twisted figment of my imagination. I squeezed my eyes shut, digging my nails into my palms, willing the ceiling tiles to melt away. But when I opened them again reluctantly, the strange room remained.

Exhaustion tugged relentlessly at the frayed edges of my mind until I could resist no longer. I curled into a tight ball atop the blankets as if making myself smaller could protect me from the world outside this cocoon. My eyes drifted shut as my mind raced wildly, unable to slow its frenetic pace.

I spiraled into a heavy sleep, but there was still no escape - only more twisting dreams of desperately running through dark woods with unseen pursuers at my heels. I jolted awake, heart hammering as I bolted upright in the strange bed. I could not slow my gasping breaths or racing pulse for long minutes, the dream's ghostly tendrils still clinging to me. As reality filtered back in, I registered two figures hovering nearby. One in scrubs - a nurse, I belatedly grasped. Beside her, Larry regarded me steadily, a crease between his brows.

"Welcome back, Elisa," the nurse began gently. Back from where? I wanted to ask. But my tongue remained leaden, mind still murky.

"You're at Mission Hospital," she continued, reading my unspoken question. "You were pretty out of it when you came in last night. We gave you something to help you rest - you've slept almost 14 hours."

Fourteen hours? I turned this over sluggishly, trying to marry it with my fragmented memories. Larry added kindly, "Josh and Tyler are fine with Mary and Tom at home. No need to worry."

My children. A fresh wave of anguish rose in me at the thought of them seeing me like this. But even that pain felt oddly muted as if filtered through gauze.

"Dr. Fields will be in shortly to evaluate you," the nurse informed me. Before I could form any reply, the two figures receded, the door clicking softly closed behind them.

I laid back against the pillows, the short exchange depleting the little energy I'd recovered. Nothing made sense yet in my fog-shrouded mind. I grasped only that I was in a hospital, being held for unknown reasons I could not yet recall or comprehend.

I drifted in and out, minutes or hours passing uncounted, until jolted alert by the door abruptly swinging open again. I blinked against the brightness as a tall, vaguely distinguishable figure entered. Dr. Fields, my sluggish brain supplied unhelpfully.

"Good morning, Elisa." The voice sounded far away, barely piercing the fog cocooning me. I tried to respond, but my tongue remained leaden, words trapped inside my head.

A penlight flashed across my vision painfully, searing brightness. I reflexively recoiled from the blinding intrusion. As my vision adjusted, blurry features resolved into a frowning middle-aged man seated beside the bed, observing me intently.

"No need to be afraid; you're safe here," he soothed. Was I afraid? I wasn't sure I was capable of feeling anything at all in this void. His mouth kept moving, more incomprehensible sounds spilling out.

"Panic...psychosis...dissociative state..." Only disjointed words penetrated before floating away again. "Medicate...keep you comfortable..."

Comfortable. The concept seemed as nonsensical and irrelevant as everything else swirling around me. I had not decided if this place was my sanctuary or my prison. Perhaps it did not matter - nothing felt confirmed in this muffled, muted realm where all edges had been softened away.

Gradually, I became aware of the doctor's expectant gaze on me. He had asked a question, I realized dimly. But the words had dispersed into the fog, their meaning lost. He tried again, more gently this time. "Are you still feeling frightened, Elisa?"

Frightened. My sluggish brain grasped at the word. Had I been frightened? Flickers of terror, that primal urge to flee, pushed through the heavy curtain shrouding my mind. Wordlessly, I managed a slight nod.

"All right. We'll get you something to help you feel calmer." He patted my hand with a professional detachment I scarcely registered before rising to leave.

My head drooped back to the pillow, his voice drifting away again. Help you feel calmer as if emotions could be controlled by dispensing pills, rationally calculated and measured. I would have laughed if I could only summon the energy.

Instead, I let my eyes fall closed again, retreating into the void where understanding remained frustratingly elusive. There was a needle prick on my arm, the creeping cold of IV drugs entering my veins, carrying me back down into heavy, dreamless sleep. A blank void where no danger could reach me because nothing felt real.

When awareness surfaced again, unsure how much time had passed, I opened my eyes to familiar faces hovering over the bed. My husband Drew, fatigue carving lines around his eyes, managed a wan smile. Behind him, Josh and Tyler peered uncertainly at me. A fresh wave of grief and remorse suffused me at my boys seeing their mother like this. Though still muted as if behind glass, the emotion cut through the buffering haze slightly.

Drew's hand on mine anchored me further, slowly tethering me back to reality. But the heavy drape still muffled my senses, time flowing past in a disconnected jumble. More clinical questions were asked gently by a revolving cast of nurses and doctors, always accompanied by the scratch of pen on the clipboard.

Once there was Larry again, his steady presence briefly penetrating the fog. And later, Drew, squeezing my hand, murmured words I could not decipher. Sometimes, there was a different bed in a different room. Injections that made the world go soft and liquid, dissolving the questions I could not answer anyway.

Gradually, incrementally, the fog lifted. Enough to understand where I was, to tentatively recount disjointed snippets of what had landed me here. But comprehension came only in hazy fragments, entire swathes of time missing from my memory. The whole truth remained submerged, shrouded in clouds I could not yet part.

I knew only that I had arrived here alone and terrified, propelled by a blind, primal instinct I did not recognize in myself. And that now

I was expected to stitch the ragged shards of my mind back into some semblance of normalcy that was perhaps forever beyond my grasp. For in the void, I had glimpsed the cracks and fissures at my very foundation. My inner architecture was profoundly, irreparably unstable.

I had stood trembling at the precipice, gazing into the churning abyss of madness. Then, take the dizzying plunge downward, unable to halt my sickening free fall. Now I was stranded alone, the climb back to solid ground stretching endlessly before me. The world I returned to looked the same, yet felt fundamentally altered. Or perhaps my perception had shifted, exposing flaws I could no longer ignore.

Either way, I would not see what I had witnessed in the darkness. No unlearning my hidden fragility laid bare. I could not step back through the doorway to the world I'd left behind. There was only moving ahead now, navigating my fractured mind the best I could.

I was irrevocably changed, staring back at my reflection as though at a stranger. My old life and self-had crumbled away, the pieces scattered beyond retrieval. Yet somehow, impossibly, I would need to gather these broken fragments and rebuild. Start again from the rubble.

For now, though, I endured. Allowed the doctors and nurses to shepherd me gently through the required motions until I was deemed fit to rejoin the world. Each day solidified a bit more from haze to reality. Each night still brought troubling dreams, but they no longer consumed me.

And so, I complied wordlessly with the pills and therapy sessions intended to restore stability. All the while knowing down to my marrow, I was now a bomb with the fuse lit. Even once discharged, it was only a matter of time until the doubt and dread crept back in. Until the kindling of my fevered thoughts ignited once more, promising to incinerate all I held dear.

The question was not if the darkness would return to claim me again. It was when. And whether I would find my way back to the light next time.

CHAPTER 3

IN THE DARKNESS

The lights in the hospital hallway seemed very bright, assaulting my senses as they led me from the intake area. I blinked against the glare, feeling dazzled and off-balance. The nurse kept up a stream of soothing chatter as we walked, but her words blurred together into meaningless background noise.

My steps faltered when we reached the room where I'd be staying. Reluctantly, I allowed her to usher me inside, my eyes darting around the barren space. The walls and floor were an icy, sterile white that gave no warmth. A simple bed with a thin mattress was pushed against one wall, an empty chair in the corner its only companion.

A wave of despair washed over me, threatening to pull me under. This was to be my sole refuge, but it offered all the comfort of a cell. I stood frozen as the nurse gave my arm a gentle squeeze.

"I know everything seems frightening right now, but we're going to take good care of you," she assured me. Her tone was kind, but the words rang hollow. She couldn't possibly understand the yawning black hole opening within me. A void this place could never fill.

"Try to get some rest. The doctor will be in to see you soon." With that, she slipped away, the door clicking decisively behind her. I listened to the echo of her footsteps disappearing down the hall until silence engulfed me.

The stark emptiness of the room was suffocating. I perched awkwardly on the edge of the creaky mattress, afraid to disturb the neatly tucked sheets. Unsure what to do with myself, I stared at my hands, twisting tightly in my lap.

The panic that had consumed me earlier was temporarily muted, pressed down by a crushing despair. My mind replayed all that had transpired in a dizzying loop - the sleepless nights consumed by fear, the panicked flight from unseen threats, and finally, the sheer terror of being pursued.

None of it felt fully real, like scenes from someone else's nightmare. Yet here I was, locked away in this cold, sterile room. A prisoner or a patient? I wasn't sure which role had been assigned to me yet.

Fatigue tugged relentlessly at my mind and body, draining the last bit of manic energy. I kicked off my shoes and curled onto the thin mattress, seeking solace from the lonely reality of this place in sleep's fleeting embrace. Yet even unconsciousness offered little respite. Feverish dreams of being trapped in a maze, pursued by faceless horrors, plagued me. Each time I reached a dead end, I jolted awake in panic, only to find myself back in the same small room. But even unconsciousness provided little respite. Feverish dreams of being trapped in a maze pursued by faceless horrors plagued me. Whenever I reached a dead end, I would jolt awake in a panic to find only the same small room.

As pale dawn light seeped through the window, I felt scarcely more rested than the night before. Exhaustion permeated every cell, yet sleep still eluded me. Every creak or footstep from the hall sent a shock of adrenaline through my system.

The door swung open suddenly, startling me. My heart pounded as I shrank back against the wall, watching warily as an orderly entered with a breakfast tray. He deposited it on the chair without a word, then departed as abruptly as he had appeared. I stared numbly at the food I had no appetite for. The pills beside the plate were indeed meant to stabilize me, but the idea of dulling my senses further was unbearable. They would remain untouched, my small act of defiance.

As the minutes ticked by sluggishly, I retreated into my thoughts. I longed desperately for someone familiar to anchor me amidst the chaos. My husband's comforting presence, or even a phone call with my mother's soothing voice. But I was isolated, cut adrift in this sterile place with no lifeline to cling to.

When the doctor arrived later to ask detached questions, I could manage only monosyllabic responses, my voice rusty from disuse. His calm, clinical demeanor offered no reassurance or comfort, just another reminder of my aloneness.

That initial day set the tone for what felt like an eternity. Time lost all meaning amidst the unchanging fluorescent lights and repetitive hospital routines. Orderlies came and went on irregular schedules, their faces blurring together. Periodically, a doctor or nurse would appear, asking questions to which I had no answers.

Once, I was moved to a different room after admitting a new patient. But nothing distinguished one cell-like space from the next. Alone on the thin mattress, I stared at yet another speckled ceiling, just like all the others.

At times, panic would surge in my chest, threatening to break the suffocating silence. Yet, the spells always passed, leaving me hollowed out and numb once more. I yearned for the nurses' comings and goings, as they were proof that a world existed beyond these claustrophobic confines. Food trays appeared randomly, though I rarely managed more than a few bites. Nothing could penetrate the choking despair muffling all emotions. Only the headaches gave me something to feel as they pounded behind my eyes, fueled by too little sleep and sustenance.

I lost track of how often the sun rose and set behind the barred window. Time ceased to flow steadily, dripping instead in sporadic drips and drabs. Every minute felt endless, yet entire hours vanished without notice. Outside that window, life went on without me - but here, I was frozen, detached utterly from any sense of normalcy.

My emotions were muted, wrapped in cotton like a comatose patient under heavy sedation. Each day brought only pale echoes of the hysteria that had landed me here. But neither did any glimmer of hope or clarity penetrate the fog.

I spent long stretches staring at the speckled ceiling tiles, accompanied by the distant hums and beeps that formed the hospital's soundtrack. The noises blended into a mechanical din, becoming the most constant companions of my days. The only reminder that I hadn't been entirely abandoned was the sporadic presence of the staff. However, even those brief interactions depleted the little energy I could summon. Instead of welcoming connections, I began to perceive them as disruptions to the fragile numbness enveloping me. Once, after yet another restless night, I woke to find my husband's concerned face peering down at me. The sight sent a fresh jolt of anguish through my chest. Seeing him in this place made my fractured mental state undeniably real rather than the nightmare I still clung to believing it was.

I could tell the stark hospital room pained him, too, hurting for my suffering. When he reached tentatively for my hand, I nearly recoiled from the tender touch. Physical contact felt dangerous, threatening to crack through the tenuous numbness and unleash a torrent of emotions I was not ready for.

But I remained still, allowing him to wrap my icy hand in his warmer one. Neither of us spoke as we sat in pained silence, the space between us filled with all the things we could not voice aloud. He looked utterly helpless watching me like this, adrift and unable to reach me.

After he left, part of me ached to call him back, yearning for the comfort of his solid presence. The rest recoiled from any reminder of the world outside. Out there, I was damaged, crazy. But cocooned here, I could pretend none of it was real.

The next time the doctor made his rounds, I asked numbly when I could go home. He gave a noncommittal response about ensuring the medication had taken effect. Inwardly, I screamed in frustration even as I maintained a passive facade.

No magic pill could mend my splintered psyche or halt the relentless waves of fear and paranoia. No amount of time in this sterile place would return me to some baseline of normalcy. But I did not have the strength to argue, so I nodded deferentially.

Later, I crept over to test the door, irrationally confident it would be locked even though I was not a prisoner. The knob turned quickly, but I left it closed. Where could I possibly go when the only place waiting for me was a home now haunted by the ghosts of who I used to be? There were no good options, only layers of confinement. Whether here or out there, loneliness and despair remained inescapable. That night, I dreamt of being trapped in an endless maze no matter how many turns I took. When an exit seemed to appear ahead, the walls would reform themselves into another dead end. Frantically, I raced through the shifting labyrinth but could not find my way out.

I awoke sobbing and shaking, the cruelty of the dream hitting too close. Because I was trapped here in this maze of my broken mind, stumbling down identical empty corridors that never led to the light. I could see no linear path forward, no way to emerge whole and stable again. Only eternal darkness, whichever way I turned.

The next day, I asked again when I could leave. This time, the doctor reluctantly said tomorrow if I remained calm. I nodded, retreating into my thoughts. After one more round of sleeping and waking in this place, the door would open again.

Would I be ready? I did not know how to answer that. Leaving here would not magically transport me back to the life violently derailed. Nothing could undo the damage done to my mind or the frightened eyes of my family.

In some ways, the hospital provided a haven from facing that harsh reality. I did not have to confront the impossibility of resuming normalcy within these walls. I could remain in stasis, sealed away from expectations and pressure.

And yet, I could not hide here forever. Time would continue flowing forward no matter how desperately I clung to the illusion that it had frozen for me in this place. The world kept turning relentlessly while I remained trapped in endless, repeating loops of my own tortured psyche.

Soon, I would have to leave this sterile cocoon and step back into that ceaselessly spinning reality. My head lifted from the shifting sands for too long; the changes that had overtaken it in my absence would be disorienting. I would emerge weakened, just as life demanded more strength than before.

The hospital had contained the crises but offered no cure for the underlying fragility in my foundations. I still felt hollowed out inside, clinging to a numb state of shock and denial. At any moment, the delicate pretense could shatter again under the pressure of routines and expectations.

Thus, I found myself suspended between the dread of rejoining the world and the desperation to escape the confines of this place. Neither option promised comfort or salvation. I struggled to convey to the doctors that while the panic had abated, the fault lines remained beneath the surface, poised to fracture at the slightest disturbance. All I could manage was a compliant nod to signal readiness for discharge, even as internal tremors betrayed my true feelings of unpreparedness. The regimented hospital days had stripped away any semblance of agency I once held. I could only defer to the doctors' judgment, incapable of advocating for myself. The next day, I rose and dressed mechanically in the clothes my husband had dropped off. I'd longed for fresh air and freedom from these claustrophobic confines for days. Now, as I awaited my release, the sterile walls provided cold comfort. Each minute brought me closer to the yawning unknown looming outside.

Too soon, there was a knock at the door before it swung open, revealing the nurse's expectant face. It was time. Woodenly, I followed her down the brightly lit halls, each step catapulting me closer to the chaos I had no tools to manage.

I kept my eyes down as we navigated through the discharge room, unable to meet the gaze of the doctor signing my release papers. As if avoiding eye contact could prevent me from seeing the doubt, the unspoken question of whether I could hold myself together outside these walls.

I took the prescriptions and instructions he had placed in my hand. Then the double doors swung open, sunlight momentarily blinding me. I froze, paralyzed by the immensity of the world awaiting me.

With a steadying breath, I compelled my leaden feet to propel me forward across the parking lot. Each step away from the hospital loosened its grip on me fractionally yet left me more untethered and exposed. I did not look back; afraid I might falter and turn around again if I did.

Though my physical body had departed the hospital, its influence lingered in unseen ways. I still felt its presence in the afterimages behind my eyes, akin to staring at the sun for too long. It echoed in the silence within, impervious to the chatter and noise of everyday life. Outwardly, I had escaped the confines of that place. Its sterile white walls and antiseptic smells were behind me. Yet, they had infiltrated my psyche, leaving a stain-like mildew that resisted easy eradication. Desperately, I clung to the fragile status quo, trusting it to bear my weight. But already, I could feel the cracks spreading beneath my feet. Fissures through which madness could come pouring in again without warning. The fall had fundamentally destabilized me, my jagged edges now exposed.

I was on the outside now but still balanced precariously on my precipice. It was only a matter of time until the next fissure cracked open, sending me back into the terrifying abyss of my mind. There would be no escaping the inevitability of that fall.

CHAPTER 4

28

A FLICKER OF HOPE

The familiar sight of our modest beige house should have been comforting. Instead, trepidation curled in my gut as Drew pulled into the driveway that first day back from the hospital.

The doctors had discharged me, deeming me recovered enough to resume life at home. But I knew the fissures were still spiderwebbing. My psyche could rupture again without warning. The home was meant to be a sanctuary, but it felt more like a stage where I'd be unable to hide the lingering damage.

With leaden steps, I moved up the walkway lined with my faded geraniums - now dried and withered after neglect. Their current state seemed an ominous sign of what else my absence had wrought.

My hands shook as I unlocked the front door, bracing for the reproachful silence. Instead, I was enveloped by welcoming warmth - the cozy furnishings, framed family photos, and even the lingering scent of cinnamon from a candle burned long ago.

For a moment, it felt as if the past weeks had been a terrible nightmare. I dared to hope that my unbroken life awaited me here.

My brief reverie shattered with the sound of footsteps. Two exuberant boys barreled into my arms, nearly bowling me over with the force of their relief.

At the sight of my children's overjoyed faces, the emotions I'd bottled up in the hospital came bursting forth. Tears streamed down my cheeks as I clung to their solid warmth.

Over their heads, my eyes met Drew's as he stood surveying the scene, tension etched across his features. In his strained gaze, I glimpsed the arduous road ahead again. The joyful reunion was a balm for now, but the wounds lurked just below the surface.

That evening, after I'd tucked the boys into bed with extra stories and kisses, their even breathing filling the quiet house, I found Drew waiting for me downstairs Without a word, he enfolded me in his strong embrace as if he could hold our broken pieces together through sheer force of will.

I allowed myself to collapse against him, soaking in the comforting solidity of his presence. Yet I felt irreparably altered even here in the circle of his arms. Like a stranger in my home, an imposter trying to blend in.

"I'm so glad you're back," Drew finally murmured into my hair. I nodded mutely against his chest, unable to voice my fears that part of me would remain forever lost in those cold hospital walls.

Sensing my inner turmoil, Drew gently guided me to sit beside him on the sofa. He stroked my hair back from my face, his eyes filled with concern and helplessness.

"I can't imagine how difficult this has been for you," he began haltingly. "I wish I could wave a magic wand and make it all disappear. But I'm here for you, no matter what you need."

I leaned into his tentative embrace, craving his strength and stability like a life raft in churning waters. Yet doubts crept in, poisoning this temporary peace.

He couldn't possibly understand how unmoored and fundamentally shaken I felt. Our lives had diverged from their familiar shared path, leaving me to traverse this treacherous terrain alone.

Nor could his steadfast support solve the underlying fissures still twisting through my psyche, threatening to rupture again at any time. However devoted, Drew was powerless in the face of my defective mind's broken wiring.

Over the following days, I clung to simple routines - preparing meals in the comforting clatter of dishes and tucking in the boys each night. Drew remained a constant, reassuring presence, watching this fragile equilibrium even as he walked on eggshells to avoid provoking another crisis.

His wariness stung, even as I understood its necessity. I was a bomb that had already detonated once, leaving only uncertainty about when or how violently I might explode again.

One evening, as we sat across from each other, picking at our dinner, the weight of all we were not saying pressed down unbearably. Desperate, I reached for his hand, anchoring myself against the doubts swirling around us.

"I'm trying...I need...time," I choked out ineptly. Time to accept my diagnosis and its lifelong implications. Time to readjust to carrying the burden of this illness. And it's time for the tentative trust between us to regrow.

Drew cradled my hands gently, his eyes overflowing with too many emotions to name. Sadness, fear, and above all, a bone-deep weariness at the prospect of weathering the unpredictable storms my condition could unleash.

"However long it takes, I'm not going anywhere," he promised solemnly. And I knew without doubt the unwavering truth of his words. But promises alone could not bridge the yawning chasm the past weeks had opened.

As the days passed, we settled into an uneasy rhythm. During moments of normalcy, I could envision our path forward together. But my darkest thoughts always came creeping back in - the insidious whispers that I was irretrievably broken, a burden he could only endure out of obligation.

Too often, I caught Drew observing me with thinly veiled worry when he thought I wasn't looking. His concern was written in the creases lining his forehead and the tight set of his shoulders.

One evening, the boys were chattering boisterously about their Little League team, but their vitality only underscored my instability. Their innocent voices blurred into shrill cacophony, every burst of laughter and scrape of silverware amping up my agitation.

Without warning, I slammed my water glass down too hard, shards scattering across the table. Shocked silence descended as four sets of startled eyes fixed on me.

"Sorry...I can't...too much..." I stammered before lurching up and fleeing upstairs to the sanctuary of the quiet bedroom. Behind me, their worried murmuring rose, grating against my raw nerves.

After several minutes, footsteps sounded tentatively on the stairs before Drew appeared in the doorway. I kept my back to him, awash in humiliation and self-loathing at losing control again.

Wordlessly, he came to sit behind me, enveloping me in his embrace. I resisted only for a moment before letting myself melt against him, taking solace in the steady rhythm of his heart beneath my ear.

"It's going to get easier," he soothed. I nodded mutely, yearning desperately to believe him. Yet the truth lurked beneath every tranquil surface - no amount of time or love could permanently banish the demons always crouching in wait inside me.

Still, it was enough to cling to Drew like ballast at this moment, keeping me from washing away in the storms. His unwavering constancy helped quiet the static in my head, keeping me tethered until I could regain my composure.

By tacit agreement, we avoided acknowledging these flare-ups once they had passed. Lingering only dredged up pain we both wished could remain buried.

But denial did nothing to fortify my crumbling foundations when the next fissure split open without warning. Little triggers ambushed me when my defenses were down, such as a sharp noise, a minor conflict, or even just the overwhelming rhythms of daily life. Drew was there to sweep up the pieces left behind each time carefully. Yet I sensed his faith fraying under the onslaught of my unraveling with its relentless aftershocks. We both threw every ounce of energy into rebuilding, but the ground never felt solid beneath me for long.

No matter how tightly I grasped the mirage of normalcy on my good days, the ever-present threat of slipping backward hung over everything. My mind had turned traitor, and nothing could force it to relent.

The boys remained bright, their joyful presence grounding me in the moment. I found peace in losing myself in their routines. Bedtime stories and school projects gave a welcome sense of purpose that my derailed plans no longer provided.

But even mothering grew challenging as my patience fluctuated wildly. On bad days, their rambunctious energy gnawed at my raw nerves until I thought I might scream. Though mostly I managed to restrain the urge, occasionally my fraying composure slipped, a harsh word escaping before I could catch it.

The wounded, confused look in their eyes in those moments was almost worse than the episodes themselves. I hated that no matter how fiercely I tried to protect them, the fallout still seeped insidiously into their lives.

Watching my children tiptoe around me was agonizing. Their childhood should have been carefree, not weighed down by their mother's terrifying instability. I had become the embodiment of all I wished to shield them from.

Each time, I resolved to do better, fighting desperately for normalcy. But despite my white-knuckled grip, it remained elusive. No amount of willpower could rein in my traitorous brain.

Medication muted the highs and lows slightly but brought a bone-deep fatigue. I slogged through days wrapped in lead, longing for relief yet terrified of lowering my defenses enough for the demons to charge through. It was an impossible dilemma.

Through it all, Drew remained steadfast by my side, my rock amidst the turbulence. But even bedrock can be worn down eventually by relentless crashing waves. The strain on him was evident in the new silver strands at his temples and the grooves lining his forehead.

Watching helplessly as I spiraled further from the woman, he married hurt him profoundly. He patiently picked up each piece I broke, even as the glue seemed to lose adhesion more rapidly each time.

When my mother gently suggested an inpatient program, I recoiled violently, seeing it as a failure. It is as if trying hard enough should be enough to patch over the fractures permanently. But deep down, I understood her logic even as I rejected it vehemently.

A gulf had opened up, separating me from the person I was before. I balanced precariously on the edge, buffeted by winds threatening to knock me over into the void. Each gust eroded my tenuous grip until, finally, my stubborn pride gave way.

When I whispered to Drew about pursuing intensive treatment, the naked relief and hope on his worn face cut me to the core. I realized he had been waiting for me to make this admission, yet unable to force the decision himself.

"Whatever it takes, we're going to get you healthy again," he promised, taking both my hands in his. His unwavering faith that the woman he loved remained was the only thing keeping me going. I prayed his stubborn optimism was not misplaced.

The first step on a new path loomed, terrifying in its immensity. But allowing someone else to steer my runaway mind temporarily offered the only glimmer of light piercing the darkness.

I eyed the long road ahead fearfully. But for the first time, I sensed a purpose beyond merely surviving daily. Where it led, I did not know. The only certainty was that turning back was no longer an option.

My hands trembled as I signed the intake forms the following day, finalizing the monumental surrender of control. As an orderly wheeled me towards the ward, I glanced back at Drew one last time.

His steadfast, loving gaze said it all. We would walk this path side by side wherever it took us. And together, we could return to the light through the darkest nights.

CHAPTER 5

35

WEATHERING THE STORMS:

The simple routines of daily life seem innocuous enough. But for me, once familiar scenes often transform abruptly into a minefield of potential triggers lying in wait. My psyche remains balanced on a knife's edge, the slightest disturbance threatening to topple me back into the abyss.

Like when the boys and I were grocery shopping - that mundane family chore suddenly morphed into psychological warfare. We walked down the canned goods aisle as the boys tossed items in the cart, their playful banter washing over me. Then, a can be dropped loudly to the linoleum, the sharp noise ricocheting through my skull. I froze, pulse instantaneously skyrocketing. A hush fell over my sons, eyeing me warily, attuned to these precarious mood shifts. I swallowed hard, fighting to steady my breathing against the surging panic. "It's okay, just startled me," I attempted brightly. Their young faces betrayed lingering unease as we resumed our routine.

But my skin still crawled with the aftershocks of adrenaline, nerves reverberating from that innocuous stimulus. A stark reminder that my brain misinterprets harmless input as dire threats, leaving me constantly warring against my defective circuitry.

On the surface, I appear whole, but inside, I ricochet endless false alarms, keeping me on high alert. Life becomes an exhausting gauntlet demanding vigilance against my volatile nature, lying in ambush around each corner.

On other days, simply bearing the onslaught of everyday family chatter becomes unendurable. The lively, overlapping voices that should seem comforting amplify unbearably in my head.

Even the compelled smile I paste on like a mask feels strained as I withdraw further into myself, muscles taut with the effort of enduring an assault upon my senses.

When it grows overwhelming, I escape under the pretense of completing some household tasks. I huddled alone in the laundry room, battling irrational irritation toward my beloved family. Their innocence makes my reaction seem all the more monstrous.

The guilt weighs on me, adding to the unbearable pressure. I should feel grateful for the everyday joys other people celebrate effortlessly. But instead, I find myself recoiling, unable to embrace the moments my traitorous mind contorts into suffering.

On my darkest days, no place feels safe from potential ambush by my psyche. Home becomes not a sanctuary but a minefield of anxiety-provoking triggers lying in wait to confirm how broken I remain.

Through it all, I strive desperately to shield Drew from the aftershocks. He handles so much already - I wish to avoid burdening him further if possible. But concealment breeds distance, which fractures fragile bonds.

So, I swallow back harsh words before they escape, pasting on a smile to hide my inner turmoil. After incidents, I downplay lasting effects, claiming to shake them off quickly. But I know he hears the truth in what I leave unsaid.

Watching me suffer shreds Drew up inside. He hides it under gentle patience, but I've caught his pained expression when he thinks I'm not looking. My instability weighs on him as heavily as on me, if not more.

His steadfast loyalty persists despite it all. On days when I cannot rise from bed under the oppressive fog smothering all motivation, he takes over parenting duties without a word of reproach.

Even on evenings when irrational reactions have flared, he pulls me into his arms and lets me cry out the shame and self-loathing. I do not deserve this man, yet I cling fiercely to the undeserved gift of his devotion.

But his tireless understanding has limits. Once, an argument flared from a petty disagreement, suddenly taking on a dangerous intensity. The nonsensical fight seemed to validate my inherent defectiveness, proving I was too broken for even Drew's love to redeem.

In desperation, I grabbed the car keys and fled into the night, seeking escape. I drove for hours without a destination or conscious thought beyond escaping the poison in my mind. But when I returned home, drained and contrite, he held me close in relieved silence.

We never spoke of that night again. On the surface, the status quo resumed. But an imperceptible shift had occurred, a microscopic fissure in unshakeable trust. A minor weakness that could spread, cracking foundations apart like water expanding in crevices of stone, Residual tension lingers now, even during peaceful moments. He watches me more warily, braced for the next unpredictable squall. Meanwhile, I hold back parts of myself to avoid further inflicting my storms upon him.

The distance does not prevent Drew from rising valiantly to meet each new crisis. But it takes a heavy toll on him, evident in the new lines on his face. He soldiers on, weary but resolute, nevertheless, the scars of weathering my storms remain.

Rationally, I know none of this is intentional, just collateral damage from the unforgiving nature of my illness. But irrational guilt consumes me anyway, knowing the torment my broken mind puts him through.

I promise I will do better each calm morning and be more robust. Yet every small trigger still carries the power to unmoor me without warning. My repeated failures to maintain stability weigh painfully on us both.

On darker days, distorted thoughts creep in, whispering that he would be better off without the deadweight of my illness dragging him down. I am failing him simply by remaining stubbornly tethered to someone too damaged to be a true partner.

But my love for this man is more vital than my illness's corrosive hold. As much as my instability has eroded our foundations, our connection remains tenaciously rooted. Storm-battered but still standing, unwilling to relinquish what we've built together.

In weaker moments, I question what is left to salvage. Can wounds heal when constantly reopened and still expect to knit properly? But Drew's steadfast devotion compels me to keep fighting for myself and us.

Recovery is never linear but fraught with painful backslides. Yet we weather each setback together, gradually fortifying ourselves against their power. My illness persists but holds less sway over our shared existence.

We have walked through the fire and emerged scarred but still whole. The blows life has dealt have only deepened our reservoirs of compassion and strengthened our stubborn will to endure. Together, we are far greater than the total of our battle scars.

The path forward may wind and sometimes double back on itself. But we follow it in lockstep, my hand clasped firmly in Drew's. With him, I can withstand the battering winds without losing my footing. And if he stumbles, I will be there to break his fall.

The disorder will continue testing our resilience, finding weaknesses in armor that must be continually reinforced. But we have learned to combat it as a united front, no longer allowing it to drive a wedge between us. Our love is a shelter where we wait out the passing storms, secure in the knowledge that clear skies will emerge again.

Battered, bowed, and bent but miraculously yet unbroken, we withstand.

CHAPTER 6

WINDS OF CHANGE

When news of Drew's transfer orders arrived, the timing felt serendipitous. As he broke the news over dinner, anticipation sparked through me. A chance at a fresh start, far from the ghosts hanging heavy here. After fifteen years of shuffling between bases and deployments, receiving our next marching orders from the Navy was nothing new. But this time felt different—a lifeline extended, offering hope of redemption from the weary battle to reclaim normalcy. I envisioned shedding old baggage like a second skin, emerging confident and carefree. Free of stares and whispers bandied about after my hospitalization seeped into small-town gossip channels.

Of course, logically, I knew those fantasies oversimplified reality. My illness wasn't so easily outrun, nor would historical chains release their grip so effortlessly. Forward momentum couldn't negate lingering fallout from tsunamis that had swept away the old foundations.

Yet still, the prospect of a blank canvas beckoned. Indeed, we could begin anew somewhere far away and untouched by the still-festering wounds here. Build the life envisioned long ago but derailed by my traitorous mind and its aftershocks.

By unspoken agreement, those dangerous currents ran too swift and deadly to examine closely before it was time to depart. We focused single-mindedly on the future awaiting just over the horizon, too alluring to resist despite obscured risks.

When moving day finally arrived, I surveyed our neighborhood block without regret. Leaving behind averted eyes and leading questions veiled as a concern. Let someone else inherit the weight of muted turmoil seeping through cracked windowpanes left carelessly open.

My shoulders felt lighter as we pulled slowly from the curb, putting literal and symbolic distance between ourselves and all this place now signified. The rearview mirror held only the promise of blank pages awaiting inscription of whatever future we dared picture.

We settled contentedly into the cross-country trek; retracing routes etched deeply from our nomadic military life. Like our pioneers charting destiny, striking out for parts unknown but shining with potential. No matter that it was merely another standard base assignment—in my fervent imagination, it gleamed bright with promise.

As homogenized highways and rest stops spooled out behind us, fresh possibilities unfurled ahead to replace tedious realities. Here, we would rediscover faded joy and laughter free of shadows. The boys would be free to roam without hovering storm clouds, their childhoods unblemished by scars not of their own.

I studied Drew's sharp side profile as he drove, strength etched in the determined line of his jaw. He had weathered every trial with steadfast grace, but I also glimpsed a burgeoning lightness in him. Together, we raced toward a future that almost dared you not to hope.

It hardly dampened my soaring enthusiasm when we finally steered up to quarters nearly identical to the last. This iteration could be a home reclaiming all that had been wrested away until nothing else existed except ordinariness.

I began making it so with feverish intensity, directing furniture placement to facilitate harmony and even seeking special touches to imbue personality into the blank canvas. Panes were flung open, admitting gentle breezes that seemed blessedly unburdened by troubles of the past.

Laughter came easier here with the possibility of filling spaces where once lurked shadows. Even the challenges of adjusting the boys to new schools were conquered rapidly, washed away on this flowing current buoying us gently skyward.

Until one otherwise forgettable afternoon when errands necessitated a stop at the busy commissary, amidst bustling aisles and inscrutable chatter, constantly swirling, some unseen shifts were unfurled like reverse Barometric pressure abruptly plunging, an unseen storm now gathering.

It began slowly—a conversation dying abruptly as I neared, renewed with intensified vigor once I passed. Fleeting yet unmistakable glances sliced my direction while mouths hidden behind hands moved furtively. No identifiable source for the whispers that raised gooseflesh on my arms, yet suddenly, they felt palpably present.

When mundane tasks were complete, I retreated hastily to the car, feeling exposed under watchful gaze's tangible as touch. Behind the safe buffer of windows, I gradually unclenched tight muscles as I maneuvered slowly from the lot, willing my pulse to steady.

You're being paranoid, a scornful inner voice accused. Indeed, no remarks had been uttered or intended with malice as I wished to believe. An overly defensive mind reeled from a sudden onslaught of unfamiliar stimuli until innocuous events took on sinister overtones.

Chalk it up to disruption from the recent moves, the cynic reasoned. Likely, no conspiracies brewed behind my back beyond trivial gossip about outsiders that would fade rapidly as we assimilated.

I grasped welcoming rationalizations like buoys, embarrassed already by humiliating overreactions. Of course, temporary destabilization was inevitable with drastic life changes. I would regain equilibrium once fully established in this environment.

But cold claws of doubt still scraped down my spine with the haunting certainty of eyes tracking my retreating form. And the disquieting notion that perhaps I could never outpace all that clung unrelentingly from the past.

I pushed aside intrusive unease, refusing to surrender my long-awaited fresh beginning to familiar ghosts. I had idealized unattainably; that was all. With flawed humans inhabiting any location, nowhere could exist without gossip, judgment, or petty jealousy. It was only that years cocooned in sickness had left me incapable of brushing off innocuous events as most individuals would. And perceived slights likely dwelled only within my still-paranoid psyche rather than reflecting actual occurrences.

This rocky transition would stabilize, given proper time and perspective to regain my bearings. I focused on gratitude for my husband's solid presence and joyful young sons, oblivious to storms swirling around us. Priorities centered on summoning inner resilience to withstand this necessary upheaval period before we emerged into calmer harbors.

But over subsequent days and weeks, the keen awareness of sideways glances and stilted silences persisting sang a different tune. Whispers intensified perceptibly as conjectures exchanged behind fluttering hands built layer by damning layer about the newcomers already branded apart.

Like wolves scenting weakness, they encircled warily, eager to expose any vulnerability. Their sly comments dissected my every move, seeking defects to validate suspicions and cement our status as outsiders. Too broken in ways visible only to their discerning pack mentality, with my erratic behavior cementing me irredeemably beyond the bounds of polite society.

Bewildered confusion chained me rooted in place during these bewildering social interactions. I lacked adequate script to navigate the harrowing minefield of conversations now laced with hidden explosives.

Desperate to believe myself intact and blameless, I ignored the writing on the walls, falsely reassuring myself that the threatening messages were unintended. Faulty wiring in my head transformed innocent misspeaks into slights verging on violence when no acts of war had been waged at all except those battling solely within my weary mind.

Yet relentless self-doubts slowly eroded my shaky confidence until bedrock certainty took hold that the defects dwelled not in my perception but resided within my failed psyche, laid bare under their scrutiny. My desperate charade at normalcy failed to satisfy the jury convened to judge whether I warranted this place within their ranks. Again and again, the damning verdict rang out clear—I remained damaged goods, my true nature evident to all who cared to look straight through flimsy veneers, unable to conceal the reality that I did not belong.

Fantasies of blank slates and fresh beginnings slowly dimmed then extinguished, the harsh light of examination revealing them as nothing but mirages. We had labored valiantly to outpace the trauma lying in silent wait within these walls. But in the end, no effort could outrun what had fundamentally and permanently altered me, an irrevocable truth betraying my brokenness wherever we roamed.

The wind's shifting course may propel passing ships safely beyond sight tomorrow. But all the wishful thinking could not erase the past or redeem me from its lingering damage. No geographical solution existed sufficient to resolve defects delineating my very essence. The same bitter refrain would echo wherever I traveled, exposing shortcomings that defined me as an outsider. Indeed, we had learned by now that no exit route could lead us far enough away to leave that behind.

CHAPTER 7

46

STEPS INTO THE LIGHT:

Accepting the truth of my diagnosis was a long, arduous road peppered with resistance and denial. Even after the dramatic psychotic break landed me straight in psychiatric care, part of me rejected the diagnosis. Indeed, one anomalous episode did not necessitate the ominous label now shadowing me.

In calmer moments, reason compelled me to acknowledge something fundamental had splintered. For my previously steady psyche to fracture so severely with no external catalyst indicated intrinsic instability belying the "normal" self-image I clung to.

Yet, as the weeks passed in a drugged haze, I wavered. Perhaps I merely needed rest and time for equilibrium to resume. Each incremental symptom reduction fed the persistent fantasy that full recovery awaited just around the next bend.

When even Drew gently confronted me with the necessity of maintenance medication, I bristled. Needing treatment implied irreparable brokenness. I withstood the debilitating side effects like penance; frame hollowed by restless misery yet preferring physical discomfort over confronting harsh reality.

For a time after hospital discharge, I managed to prop up a passable imitation of myself once more. The demanding rigors of parenting and maintaining a household provided an adequate distraction from my fractured state. On the surface, the woman others saw appeared nearly whole.

But behind the façade, my psyche remained splintered, scarcely held together by fraying threads and sheer stubborn will. Relentless insomnia left me hollow-eyed and worn, yet I resisted acknowledging the instability churning beneath rigid self-control. Teetering recklessly on the precipice became an acceptable status quo. Anything was preferable to admitting powerlessness.

When well-meaning psychiatrists suggested adjusting medications to alleviate still-acute symptoms, I bristled. Indeed, additional combinations exacerbating already severe fatigue would only magnify helplessness rather than reinstate control. Yet even I eventually had to acknowledge bedridden and ineffective hardly constituted durable recovery.

And so began the demoralizing trial-and-error process of navigating treatment options, balancing symptom management against devastating side effects. Every failed attempt at stability seemed to undermine my defective constitution further until even basic functionality hung tenuously in the balance.

Against these setbacks, Drew remained a steadying force - supporting but not strong-arming, despite his desperation. I discerned the toll my refusal took on him, how each downward spiral carved deeper worry lines across his forehead. But he continued delicately nudging me forward when I faltered without ever explicitly wresting control I so fiercely guarded.

When a particularly wretched medication cocktail landed me back at the hospital, reality finally penetrated stubborn denial. The cycling episodes had progressed beyond my capacity to constrain through sheer bullheadedness. Stability would remain elusive without proper maintenance to govern a mind functioning independently of my rigid directives.

The surrender of authority over my faulty psyche devastated long-held illusions of self-determination. Relinquishing that bone-deep resistance and handing over the reins felt akin to acknowledging the death of the self I had always known.

In my heart, I recognized letting go as the sole remaining path forward. Still, I grieved profoundly as Dr. Brennan cautiously reiterated the importance of maintaining medication under psychiatric supervision. Her quiet affirmation of my illness's inescapable permanence was the final nail in the coffin containing my former identity.

Numbly, I finally committed to full adherence, simultaneously crushed by this acknowledgment of lifelong affliction yet cognizant that no alternative avenues remained. After years of resisting the indignity of such constraints, weariness finally overruled pride.

I wish I could describe the subsequent breakthrough as instantaneously revelatory, but transformation unfolded gradually through a relentless slog. Together with Dr. Brennan, I continued navigating countless tweaks, seeking an elusive balance between efficacy and tolerability. Blind alleys frequently necessitated backtracking and detours when side effects overwhelmed progress.

Triumph emerged piecemeal, often two steps forward and then one step back. My perspective shifted from battling a paternalistic medical establishment to a shared mission for wellness. Healing was no longer defined solely by the absence of acute symptoms but by the cultivation of more profound wisdom and purpose.

As my interior state eventually stabilized, mental quietude replaced ceaseless inner clamor. I marveled anew at forgotten sensations - relaxing into the tranquility of unbroken sleep, embracing simple joys without bracing for the other shoe to drop. Holding lengthy conversations without losing the thread to intrusive background noise in my head. Almost miraculously, stability unlocked capacities for intimacy and insightful observation previously obscured.

Of course, vestiges of the old perspective still echo at times. Occasional intermittent side effects still trigger former tendencies toward self-blame for perceived weakness. As dopamine channels recalibrate from chemical assistance, I must battle old demons mostly silenced but awaiting any opportunity to resurrect formerly ingrained thought patterns.

Fortunately, new pathways paved through hard-fought inner work now offer alternative routes to circumvent traps I once considered inescapable. My toolbox overflows with strategies for resilience judiciously crafted over long toil. When familiar specters arise, I draw on these arsenals with the quiet confidence of an experienced warrior. My honor scars prove confrontation and endurance against the most cunning adversary I have ever faced - my beautiful brain turned traitor.

No true victory or decisive declaration of ultimate triumph remains attainable while this lifelong dance continues. But through an unrelenting warrior spirit, I can channel inevitable setbacks into springboards for growth rather than excuses for resignation or self-blame for imagined failure.

My guiding light and battle inspiration is the family who stood stalwart through long, hopeless nights when flares sparked uncontrolled wildfires and morning revealed only scorched earth. Their patient, enduring love inspired me to soldier on when no fuel remained to burn. Even if only for their sake, I would rise time and again from ashes still smoldering below the inevitable subsequent ignition.

Perhaps someday, permanent remission or a miraculous cure could manifest the unforeseen. But odds predict this partner, and I will tango endlessly to maintain fragile equilibrium commandeered off-course recklessly by a few faulty neurons. Though daunting, the exhaustive journey has forged bonfire-hot perseverance and wisdom enough to fill volumes from those who walked through the crucible still somehow emerging intact on the far side.

Now, with weathered determination, I stand squarely facing uncertain elements arrayed ahead, refusing to cede hard-claimed ground back to unseen foes determined to undermine foundational recovery. No matter how fortunes unfold in uncharted terrain unfurling ahead, I remain rooted firmly in who I fought like hell, reinstating as pilot of my destiny. Whatever healing pends or setbacks arise, I stand confident and unfaltering against gathering storms. Having stared down the beasts and beholding, my beauty reflected even from places of most profound darkness. Ready for anything, everything, absolutely nothing fazes me now.

CHAPTER 8

DARKNESS AND LIGHT:

In the stillness of the early morning, standing at my bedroom window with a coffee cup warming my palms, the world appears pristine. Anything seems possible in the quiet moments before sunrise washes yesterday's resolutions away. I inhale deeply, filling my lungs with optimism to fuel another day of grappling with unpredictable forces beyond my control.

I have learned through grueling experience that steadiness emerges not from passive expectation but relentless, active will that this too shall pass. Like a warrior, I don armor daily, fortifying myself to withstand relentless psychic attacks lurking unknown over each horizon. Tranquility is hard won, an oasis perpetually under siege requiring vigilant guarding. It could be sapped in an instant if my defenses waver.

And so, I brace for each new dawn's onslaught, having witnessed too often how rapidly the other shoe drops without warning. No matter how smoothly life may flow, I sleep with one eye open, knowing stomach-dropping disorder waits dutifully in the wings, preparing the next scheduled entrance after every graciously brief exit. One symptom recedes only for another to emerge hydra-like from stealthy depths, advancing the cyclic dance between darkness and light.

Perhaps some elusive stability may arrive in years, signaling the curtain's close on this exhausting production. But nothing etched in the historical record suggests we have seen the final act of an epic saga spanning a lifetime. I expect our pas de deux shall continue indefinitely, my reliable adversary rising boldly to challenge hard-won equilibrium through our elegant choreography predestined never to culminate in a decisive resolution.

And so we spin on, darkness and light eternally alternating dominance. At times, grief arises due to witnessing the seemingly effortless homeostasis most people inherit by mere accident of ordinary biochemistry. Resentment wells observing their blithe unconsciousness of inhabiting an intrinsic balance I fiercely battle maintaining. Surely, I deserve no less than baseline function freely afforded everyone around me by sheer luck?

But mostly, I have made peace with cards arbitrarily dealt, focusing energy on learning to play them with utmost skill to compensate for unfair advantage. If my weary challenger persists in behaving unconscionably, then so too shall I, rising to meet each new assault with equally indefatigable tenacity. Resigned to an indefinite contest between light and dark battling for supremacy within my mind, I dig in for a lifelong endurance race.

The key weapon cultivated through challenging experience is rigorous self-care, a critical bulwark defending internal equilibrium when outside forces gather into perfect storms. I carve out small sanctuaries against the relentless siege, assiduously tending these oases, providing respite and restoration between battles.

The calming evening ritual of a candlelit bubble bath transports me to a serene state, reinforcing psychic barriers. Morning meditation centers stability before commencing daily combat maneuvers. Gentle gardening connects me to larger rhythms when the inner terrain grows brutally inhospitable.

I wield fierce personalized discipline, dispelling chaos and refusing surrender. Financial safeguards ensure access to ammunition should occupations become casualties of war campaigns sabotaging functionality. Boundaries establish perimeters fortifying precious inner reserves; margin spaces open around consuming routines so their maws cannot swallow me entirely.

My secret weapon for empowering resilience is humility and acknowledging limitations. I plot pacing wisely rather than expending all firepower on isolated skirmishes. Regrouping during respites prevents fatigue, depleting ongoing stamina for prolonged engagements. I calculate risk-benefit judiciously before volunteering extra vulnerability.

When darkness inexorably reasserts its rightful place center stage, I welcome its haunting beauty now with hard-won reverence rather than futile resistance. Flowing through manic fire or depressed frozen wastelands equally expands spiritual capacities if you release a white-knuckled grip on what cannot be controlled. Meditative surrender transports me beyond mundane reality's narrow constraints into transcendent realms where meaning takes form unrecognizable to ordinary perception.

I think of the Phoenix mythic cycle of self-immolation, then rising triumphantly to regenerate from the smoldering ashes of former incarnations. We endure repeated dissolution yet emerge purified by consuming flames into more glorious, resilient versions only attained through a baptismal passage through hell realms. Darkness creates traction against which our light is thrown into majestic relief. Together, they exist in reciprocal balance, symbiotic counterweights through a gravitational dance spanning the poles of human experience.

When health crumbles under vicious internal mutiny, I remind myself this is perfection that wants to be expressed as part of inescapable unfolding. My travails serve purposes beyond visible terrain if I develop faculties perceiving broader landscapes of cause and meaning. I turned my senses toward whispered wisdom on subterranean breezes when banished to underworld domains. If darkness brings gifts, radical acceptance allows me to receive them gracefully as growth opportunities are mysteriously concealed inside adversity's gnarled shell.

And so, we waltz tirelessly, my nemesis and I, through rhythms beyond our control yet punctuated occasionally by transcendent insight. As symptoms flare and then ebb at predictable intervals, I flow intuitively through manic tidal forces. Harnessing excessive energy channeled into new pursuits and creative expressions before it inevitably recedes then restores me battered to shore, awaiting the next incoming wave.

No cure promises permanent liberation from cyclic storms forever darkening this landscape. But rescue arrives through radical acceptance of ebbs and flows as integral choreography rather than meaningless chaos to rail against futilely. Darkness strips me to the essence and then molds more muscular vessels from clay left pulverized. Each round fortifies courage and resilience for subsequent descents.

I stand naked, head raised, unflinching to howling elemental fury. My travels through infernal regions reveal that darkness contains pinpoints of light if you adjust vision to its dazzling frequencies. Just as hidden within most piercing brightness waits for corresponding pockets of impenetrable shadow. Threaded together seamlessly within a cosmic tapestry to form sublime beauty transcending human comprehension of intertwined dark and light. Two integral halves are unified into a whole.

CONCLUSION CHAPTER

My life's journey has traced a long and winding arc, filled with more twists and turns than I could have anticipated. From the first terrifying psychotic break that upended everything stable and familiar to the years of turmoil that followed, I've weathered torrential storms.

Yet somehow, through the depths of hopelessness, I discovered glimmers of light along the way. Hard-won tears of acceptance crystallized into pearls of wisdom over time. And slowly, falteringly, the clouds began to part, revealing brighter rays glowing steadily on the horizon.

The road has been anything but smooth or straightforward. Bipolar disorder made sure of that. For every step forward, another setback loomed in my periphery, threatening to derail all progress immediately. Maintaining equilibrium in such unreliable terrain felt eternally beyond my control or capabilities.

But with each relapse, as agonizing as they were, came expansions of compassion - for myself and others similarly struggling. Repeated brushes with the black veil of depression cultivated resilience and deepened my capacity to sit with suffering. Exposures to the heights of mania revealed sides of myself that, harnessed appropriately, could be channeled into extraordinary creativity.

Of course, I lacked such perspective in the beginning. The initial diagnosis felt like a crushing sentence, sentencing me to lifelong imprisonment ruled by my defective brain's whims. The medications and therapies prescribed seemed just as controlling, robbing me of autonomy over my identity and experiences. Psychiatric treatment was something forced upon me, not an empowering toolkit freely chosen from a place of self-knowledge and intention.

But that victim mentality could only sustain me so long in the face of realities refusing to bend. Bargaining and railing against the injustice of it all wasted precious energy that could be better directed toward healing.

No matter how desperately I longed to outrun this disorder, it would forever remain encoded in my DNA. The only viable option was to stop fleeing and finally turn to face it eye-to-eye.

With radical acceptance came the lightning bolt revelation that I was not solely at the mercy of unpredictable symptoms. Yes, I would likely spend a lifetime balancing periodic episodes that even optimal treatments could not fully control. My condition might wax and wane but could be counted upon to resurface periodically. Yet diagnosis did not equate to prognosis – the path of my illness did not inherently chart the path of my life.

Choice by precious choice, step by shaky step, I transitioned from reluctant passenger to empowered driver of my wellness and destiny. I surrounded myself with supportive friends who could hold space for messy imperfections. Letting go of fabulist futures, I pursued small passions that sparked joy. Gentleness and self-compassion eased harsh inner voices cultivated over the years, internalizing stigma. Forgiveness allowed healing where judgment had formerly festered. And meaning slowly accrued through attention to life's subtle graces and interconnections so often obscured when lost in inner turmoil.

In retrospect, the topography of my life appears almost fated. Each staggering blow forged more solid foundations from the rubble, like adaptive pressure transforming carbon into diamonds or winds shaping limestone's hidden beauty, adversity excavated strength and resilience that could not be cultivated any other way.

Shedding the last vestiges of self-recrimination, I realize now that psychological wounds are a necessary price. Suffering deeply expands our capacities exponentially once healed. My dance with darkness gifted perspectives and capacities for profound empathy I may not have otherwise developed in an untroubled life of smooth privilege.

My diagnosis connects me to a robust community built on radical honesty regarding mental health struggles. Together, we confront outdated stigmas and raise our voices to advocate for compassionate solutions. The unique vantage point afforded by my condition allows me to offer hope to others grappling with similarly unpredictable terrain. My story provides a beacon for terrified newly diagnosed souls, reassuring them through my example that the other side of despair holds unbelievable beauty if only they can hang on long enough.

Some mornings, the familiar weight temporarily returns as I question whether I have the strength to shoulder another episode's crushing load. But those dark moments pass as fleeting clouds cross an endless sky. Instinctual fear no longer overrides bone-deep, knowing I can and will endure whatever arises with grace and courage. Each time, I emerge a little stronger and a little wiser than before.

The future's certainty lies only in its uncertainty. My disorder may continue to ebb and surge beyond my control. But I meet each new day rooted firmly in hard-won self-acceptance, connected to sources of meaning, belonging, and purpose that transcend any diagnosis. Dark spells come and go, but inner light persists steadily now, illuminating the way forward with hope.

Mine is but one story among multitudes. Everyone faces challenges that feel, at times, beyond their capacities. But the human spirit's unbelievable resilience enables us to endure adversity and transmute it through the alchemy of wisdom and love. Darkness prevails only if we lose sight of the shared light.

As I reflect on the long road behind me, gratitude overwhelms any lingering shadows. My guiding truth now is that we all possess the power to take the broken shards life deals us with and slowly piece them into magnificent mosaics. Healing begins when we stop fighting reality's shape and start trusting in our sacred ability to construct beauty from whatever arises.

My journey has tested me to the marrow of my bones. But such ordeals reveal that flame even when compressed into a diamond. No matter what the next chapter holds, I know the light I carry within can illuminate any darkness. And for that unshakeable knowledge and the long road that led me here.